handcrafted
LIP BALMS

A MEDLEY OF ALL-NATURAL RECIPES

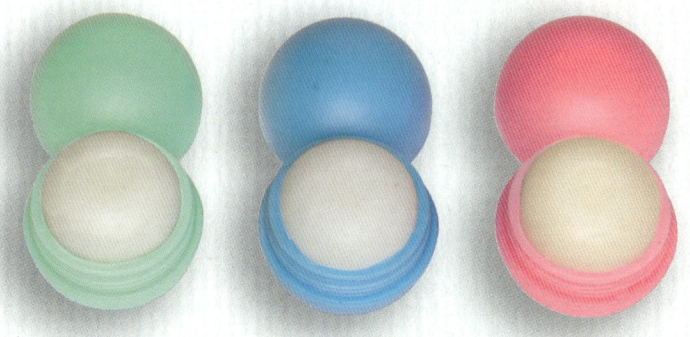

Betsy Henry Pringle
&
Nancy W. Cortelyou

becker&mayer! books

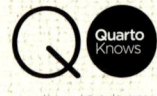

Brimming with creative inspiration, how-to projects, and useful information to enrich your everyday life, Quarto Knows is a favorite destination for those pursuing their interests and passions. Visit our site and dig deeper with our books into your area of interest: Quarto Creates, Quarto Cooks, Quarto Homes, Quarto Lives, Quarto Drives, Quarto Explores, Quarto Gifts, or Quarto Kids.

© 2018 Quarto Publishing Group USA Inc.

Published in 2018 by becker&mayer! books, an imprint of The Quarto Group.
11120 NE 33rd Place, Suite 201, Bellevue, Washington 98004.
www.QuartoKnows.com

This book is part of the *Handcrafted Lip Balms kit* and is not to be sold separately.

becker&mayer! books titles are also available at discount for retail, wholesale, promotional, and bulk purchase. For details, contact the Special Sales Manager by email at specialsales@quarto.com or by mail at The Quarto Group, Attn: Special Sales Manager, 401 Second Avenue North, Suite 310, Minneapolis, MN 55401 USA.

18 19 20 21 22   5 4 3 2 1

ISBN: 978-0-7603-6218-1

Library of Congress Cataloging-in-Publication Data available upon request.

Authors: Betsy Henry Pringle and Nancy W. Cortelyou
Interior and Package Design: Megan Sugiyama
Editorial: Betsy Henry Pringle, Paul Ruditis, and Meredith Mennitt
Production: Blake Mitchum and Shawn Reed
Photography: Chris Burrows

MIX
Paper from responsible sources
FSC® C017606
www.fsc.org

Quarto UK, The Old Brewery
6 Blundell Street, London N7 9BH, UK

Allen & Unwin
30 Centre Rd, Scoresby VIC 3179, AUS

Printed, manufactured, and assembled in Shenzhen, China, 8/18.

IMAGE CREDITS: Ann.and.Pen/Shutterstock.com, Marina Akinina/Shutterstock.com, Protasov AN/Shutterstock.com, Dmitrij Skorobogatov/Shutterstock.com, Kolomiec/Shutterstock.com, Mir141/Shutterstock.com, SOMMAI/Shutterstock.com, Alenka Karabanova/Shutterstock.com, Dariia Baranova/Shutterstock.com

305179

Contents

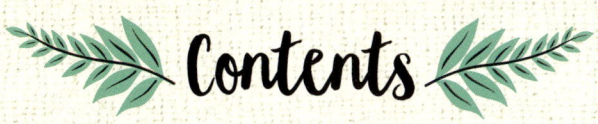

Introduction

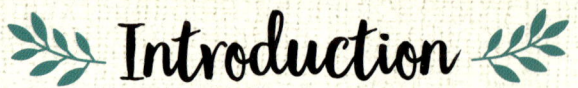

Oil and beeswax are the only ingredients you need to whip up handcrafted lip balms.

Simply melted together and allowed to cool, natural oils and waxes moisturize the skin resulting in soft, healthy lips. But why stop there? By adding simple ingredients, like chocolate chips, honey, and flavored oils—most of which are likely in your pantry—you can craft a whole array of lip balms. On their own, the suggested add-ins are fun and effective, but consider boosting your balms with more specialty ingredients like vitamin E, liquid glycerin, or castor oil for a full spectrum of colors, flavors, and benefits.

This kit includes the beeswax and step-by-step instructions to launch your creative expression. Start with these recipes, and then devise formulas of your own. Most add-in ingredients you choose to include will be stirred into the melted oil and beeswax. You'll soon have an arsenal of tried-and-true recipes.

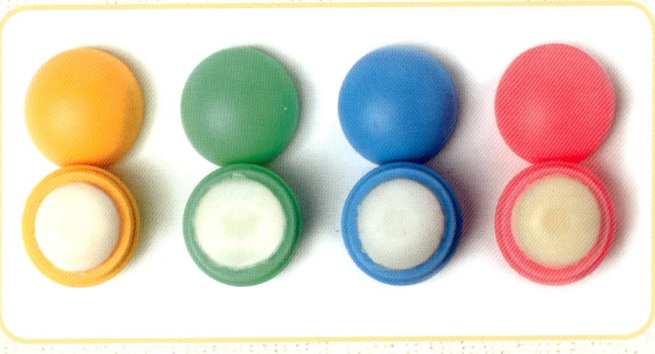

What's Included in This Kit

Inside you'll find the following materials to get started making your own lip balms:

- Beeswax pastilles (1.5 ounces/42.2 grams)
- PVC mold
- 6 lip balm pods with inserts

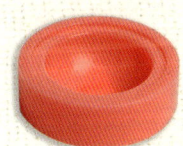

PVC Mold

POD PARTS

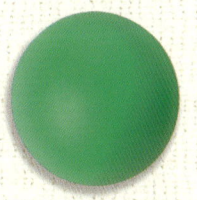

Top

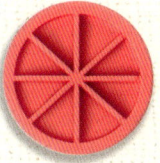

Insert

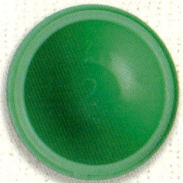

Bottom

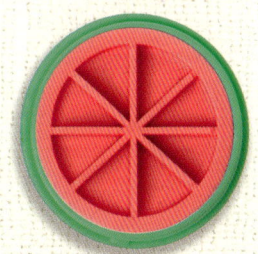

Press an insert into the bottom of a pod.

Pod parts are interchangeable. Match—or mix—the colors.

There is enough beeswax in this kit to make all of the book's lip balms, plus a few concoctions of your own. Purchase additional beeswax at craft stores or online.

Ingredients, Tools & Other Materials

There are two basic ingredients needed to make any lip balm: oil and beeswax.

BEESWAX

Beeswax works as a binder holding the lip balm's ingredients together. And because it seals in moisture, kills germs, conditions the skin, and feels wonderful, it's the perfect base for lip balms, lotions, creams, and cosmetics!

Bees produce beeswax as part of the honeycomb-building process—and humans use it for all kinds of things. Sweet-smelling beeswax has been used for embalming mummies, making candles, protecting food, and creating art.

OIL

Most of the recipes do not specify a particular type of oil. You may find a favorite that you stick with, or better yet, keep mixing it up. Experiment with any of these oils: olive, safflower, canola, corn, grape seed, sunflower, almond, or avocado. Note that extra-virgin olive oil may be too harsh in color and taste. You decide!

INGREDIENT ADD-INS USED IN THIS KIT

Once your base is mixed, create something special with one (or more) of these add-in ingredients:

Candy coloring oils: found with candy-making supplies

- Candy flavoring oils: found with candy-making supplies
- Candy melt wafers: found with candy-making supplies
- Chocolate chips
- Cocoa butter
- Coconut oil
- Cosmetic-grade glitter: found in craft stores
- Honey
- Lemon-flavored oil
- Lipstick (for color)
- Liquid glycerin: found in the first aid section of drug stores
- Chocolate hazelnut spread
- Vanilla extract
- Vitamin E capsules

> Candy coloring oils are highly concentrated, so start with the tiniest amount possible to build your desired hue. And, candy flavoring oils only require a drop or two to do the trick. Mix thoroughly.

HELPFUL TOOLS

- Microwave oven (or a double-boiler)
- 1 cup (225 mL) microwave-safe measuring cup. (A shallow coffee mug works too, but it's best to have a spout as well as a handle.)
- Blunt table knife
- Wooden stir sticks
- Measuring spoons
- Paper towels for cleanup

Tips, Techniques & Troubleshooting

DOS

- Do set up all your tools and ingredients near the microwave for easy creating.
- Do keep hot oils away from children and pets.
- Do experiment with add-in ingredients and amounts and types of oils.
- Do toss out balms after two months and make fresh ones.

DON'TS

- Don't heat oils and waxes for more than 30 seconds at a time.
- Don't add food coloring to your lip balms—it won't mix in, and the dye can rub off on your skin and clothing.
- Don't add aloe vera gel or other water-based ingredients to your recipes—they won't mix in.
- Don't add plants, herbs, or spices. Stick to oils.

FIND THE BALANCE

Getting the right balance of oil and beeswax is the key to a successful lip balm. If your lip balm doesn't glide easily, it has too much beeswax. If it feels greasy, it has too much oil. Fix it by re-melting the mixture and adjusting the ingredient amounts accordingly.

Remember, the recipes are meant to inspire your own exploration. Testing out potential ingredients in various quantities is your pathway there.

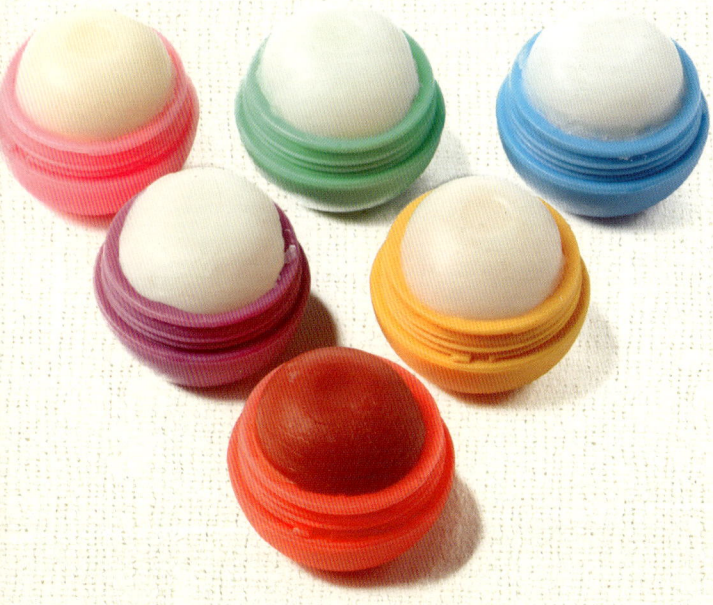

Cleanup

Waxes and oils don't mix well with water, which can make cleanup a challenge. Here are some tips for getting it done.

Between recipes: To clean a waxy cup between recipes, wipe the inside thoroughly with a paper towel (or two). It helps if the wax is still slightly warm.

Done for the day: When you're done experimenting for the day, wipe the warm wax out of the measuring cup with a paper towel. Pour some boiling water and a few drops of dish soap into the cup to melt the remaining wax. After a few seconds, pour out the water and wipe the cup clean with a paper towel. Be careful how much is going down the drain. Because wax does not dissolve in water—instead, it just hardens—you'll want to avoid getting melted wax in your sink and drains.

CLEANING INSERTS AND PODS

1. Scrape off as much waxy balm as you can.
2. Place the pod parts into a heat-safe bowl with a little dish soap.
3. Pour boiling water into the bowl.
4. When all the wax has melted, use a spoon to scoop the clean item out of the hot water.
5. Rinse off the pod parts with soap and water.

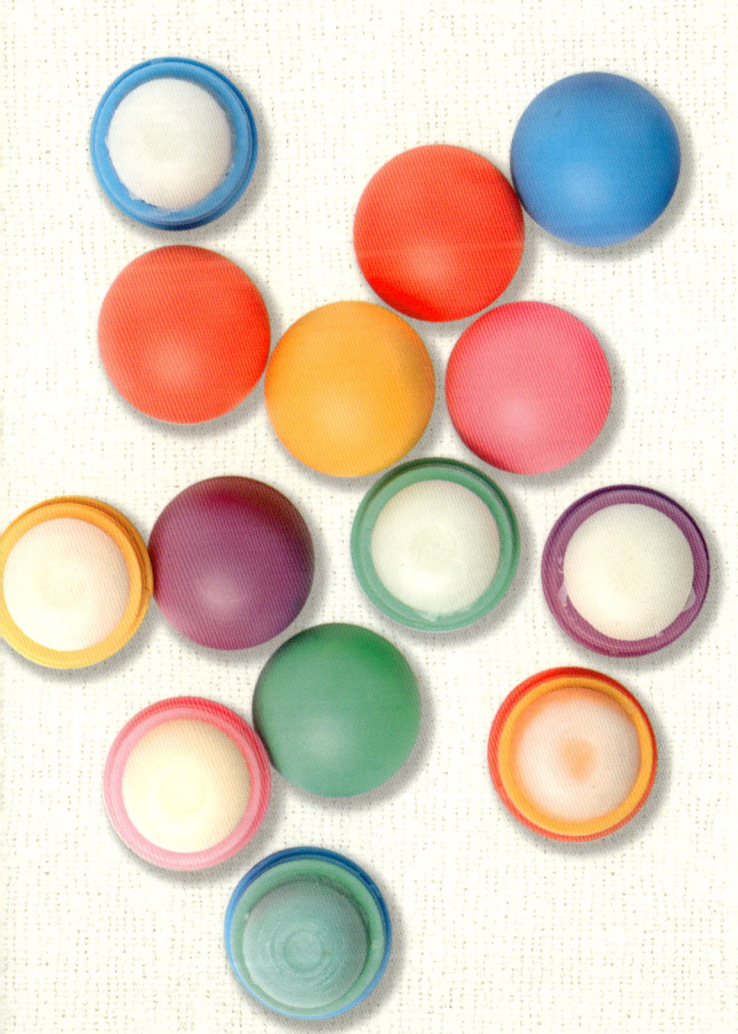

Great Moments in Lips-Story

5,000 YEARS AGO

Ancient Mesopotamian women get credit for innovating lipstick—or at least a version of it. Coating their lips with crushed semi-precious jewels, they, essentially, bedazzle their mates.

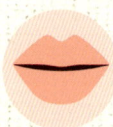

4,000 YEARS AGO

Egyptian lip stains are concocted from fungus and a highly toxic substance literally "to die for."

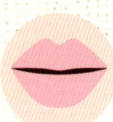

2,500 YEARS AGO

Cleopatra DIYs her own beeswax-based lip balm, adding crushed cochineal carmine beetles. The tiny bugs help her achieve a crimson color thanks to the red cactus berries they ingest. Beetles juice, as it were, is safe for most people to ingest and is still being employed in cosmetics—and food products—today.

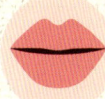

EUROPEAN DARK AGES

Lipstick is banned for a really long time.

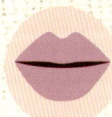

16TH CENTURY

Queen Elizabeth I resurrects lipstick during her reign, popularizing the look of dark red lips on a white face. This time around, the beeswax-based beauty tool is made from natural, plant-derived dyes. However commonplace the look is at the time, it conjures up clown makeup to the modern eye.

18TH CENTURY

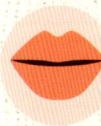

After Queen Elizabeth's I's reign ends, lipstick is again a restricted and rare cosmetic, primarily seen on the stage or in red-light districts. The British Parliament even goes as far as trying to outlaw it for single girls, claiming that it is witchcraft for luring men to marry.

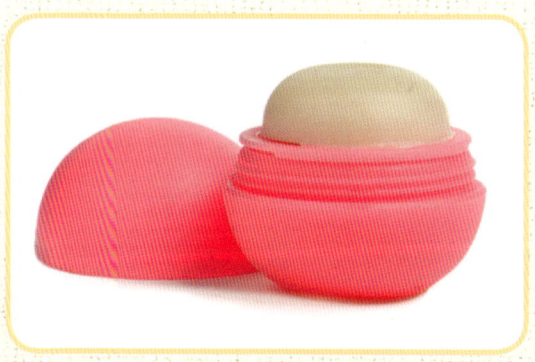

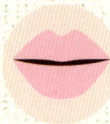

EARLY 1880S

Dr. Charles Browne Fleet invents lip balm—a recipe that ultimately becomes Chapstick—peddling it in a candle-like form wrapped in aluminum foil. But it isn't Dr. Fleet who makes it famous. After failing to make his product a success, he sells it in 1912 to a local resident, John Morton, for $5 (about $120 today). Morton and his wife cook up Chapstick in their kitchen, and the rest is history.

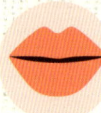

LATE 1880S

Actresses of the silent screen bring red lips back! Keen to darken their pouts to better stand out in black-and-white films, actresses use a variation of Cleopatra's mix: carmine dye taken from the scales of cochineal insects. This time the mixture is more natural looking, packaged in small pots, and applied with a brush or a fingertip.

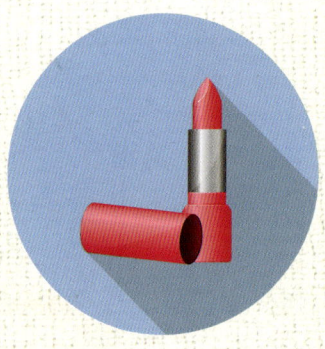

EARLY 1900S

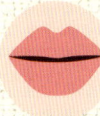

The invention of a cylindrical tube (the now-ubiquitous swivel technology would be added later) improves ease of application. The world embraces lipstick, lip gloss, and lip balms, making them mainstream lip needs.

WORLD WAR II

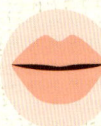

Although strict rationing is endured during the war, Winston Churchill deems lipstick to have a positive effect on wartime morale, choosing to keep it in production.

2000S

EOS revolutionizes the lip industry by taking things out of the tube and into a no-fingers-needed pod (just like those in this kit).

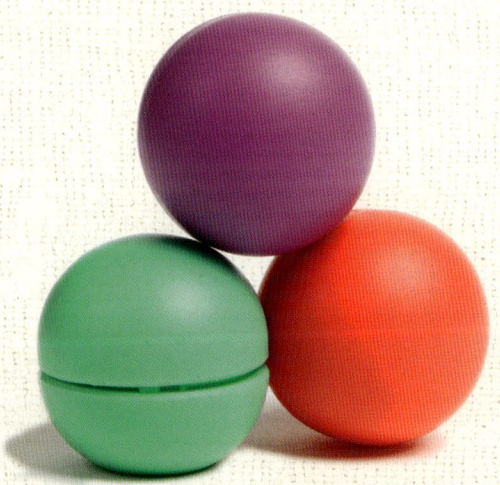

A Note About the Recipes

All of the lip balm recipes in this book call for the same two base ingredients: oil and wax. The amounts used are approximate, and meant to help you get started. Experiment your way toward the best results and new concoctions. As long as the oil and wax are in place, the sky's the limit. When you're ready to branch out on your own, use this simple formula to start:

FOR ONE LIP BALM

- 1 teaspoon (5 mL) oil
- 1/2 teaspoon (2.5 mL) beeswax pastilles
- Add-ins: stir into the melted oil and beeswax

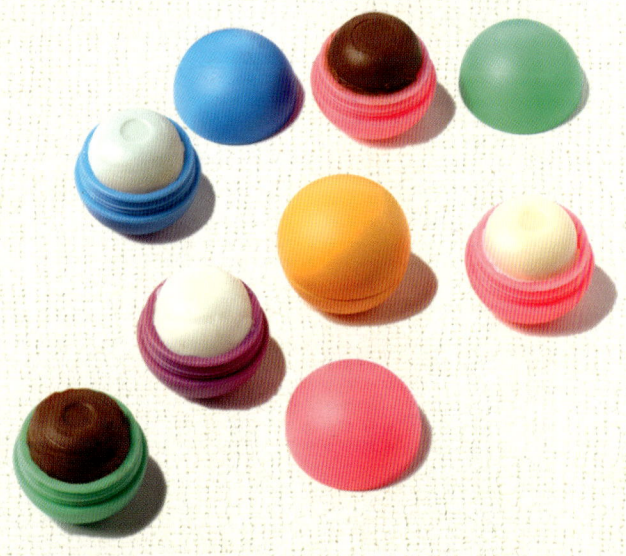

INSTRUCTIONS

1. Into a microwave-safe measuring cup, combine the oil and beeswax. Stir.

2. In a microwave oven, heat the cup for 30 seconds on high. The mixture will be hot! Stir. If the beeswax is not melted, heat the mixture in 10-second intervals, until fully melted.

3. Add the add-ins, chocolate in this case, and stir until incorporated.

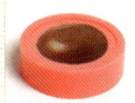

4. Pour the mixture into the PVC mold until it completely fills the sphere with a little "dome" on top. (If you overfill, you can wipe off the excess after it cools.)

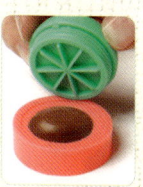

5. Wait 30 seconds, then place the insert and bottom onto the top of the melted ingredients. Let the wax harden for 25 minutes. (If you want to speed up the process, place the mold in the freezer.)

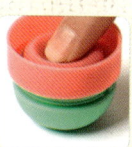

6. Gently press on the dimple in the mold to set the balm firmly into the insert. (If balm spilled over the edge when you were filling the mold, now is the time to wipe it off with a tissue.)

7. Rub your lip balm creation onto your lips! Remember to discard any unused balm after two months.

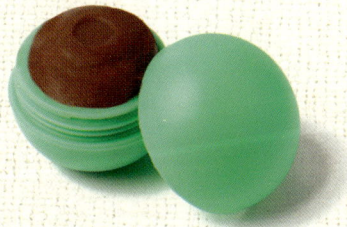

Coconut Oil Lip Balm

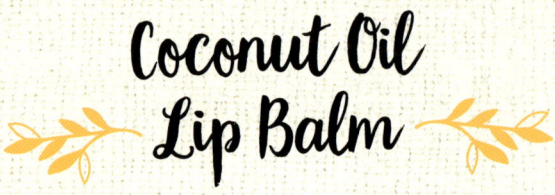

Coconut oil is derived from the meat of the coconut. It's solid at room temperature, it melts quickly into your skin. It's rich with antioxidants that fight skin irritation. Plus, it tastes delicious. In this lip balm, it is the oil of choice. No add-in ingredients needed (unless you want!).

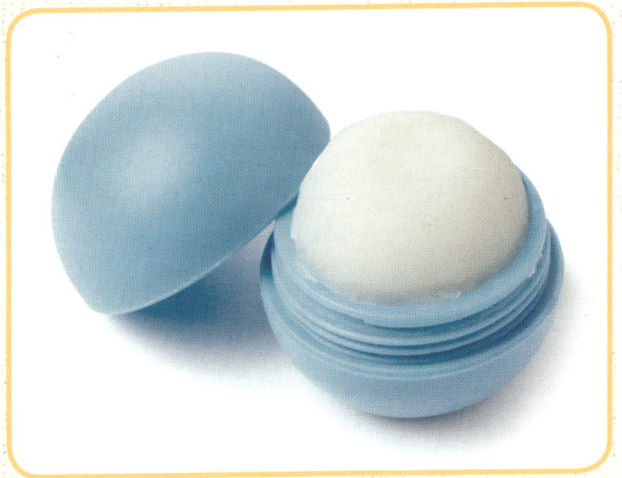

INGREDIENTS

1 teaspoon (5 mL) virgin coconut oil

1/2 teaspoon (2.5 mL) beeswax pastilles

TOOLS

Microwave-safe measuring cup

Measuring spoons

Stir stick

PVC mold (from this kit)

Pod with insert (from this kit)

MAKES ONE LIP BALM

INSTRUCTIONS

1. Into a microwave-safe measuring cup, combine the oil and beeswax. Stir.

2. In a microwave oven, heat the cup for 30 seconds on high. The mixture will be hot! Stir.

3. If the beeswax is melted, you're ready to pour. If the beeswax is not melted, heat the mixture in 10-second intervals, until fully melted.

4. Pour the mixture into the PVC mold until it completely fills the sphere with a little "dome" on top. (If you overfill, you can wipe off the excess after it cools.)

5. Wait 30 seconds, then place the insert and bottom onto the top of the melted ingredients. Let the wax harden for 25 minutes. (If you want to speed up the process, place the mold in the freezer.)

6. Gently press on the dimple in the mold to set the balm firmly into the insert. (If balm spilled over the edge when you were filling the mold, now is the time to wipe it off with a tissue.)

7. Rub your lip balm creation onto your lips! Remember to discard any unused balm after two months.

Tropical Cocoa Butter Lip Balm

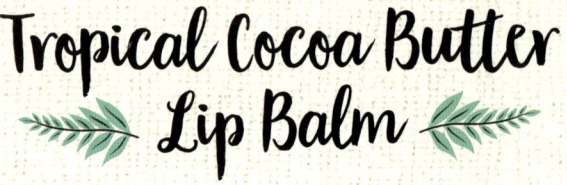

Your scent memory of cocoa butter likely conjures up the beach—or poolside days. That's because it is often mixed along with coconut in suntan lotion to achieve a tropical smell. Cocoa butter offers quick relief to dry lips, keeping skin smooth and soft with the added ability to create a barrier to outside elements that can cause irritation. Inhale the scent of the tropics with this cocoa-butter-based balm.

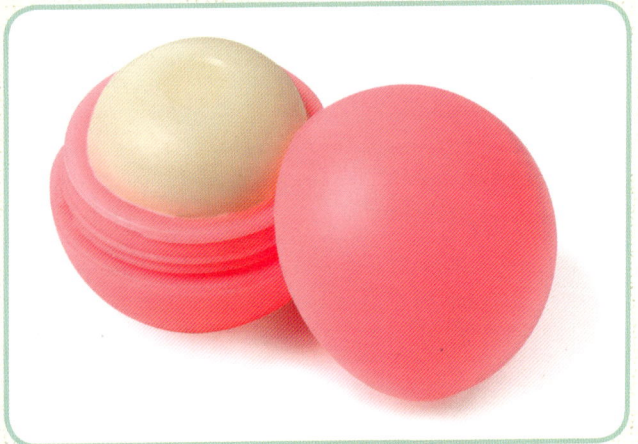

INGREDIENTS

1/2 teaspoon (2.5 mL) cocoa butter
1/2 teaspoon (2.5 mL) oil
1/2 teaspoon (2.5 mL) beeswax pastilles

TOOLS

Grater or chef's knife
Microwave-safe measuring cup
Measuring spoons
Stir stick
PVC mold (from this kit)
Pod with insert (from this kit)

MAKES ONE LIP BALM

INSTRUCTIONS

1. Grate or chop the cocoa butter into small pieces.

2. Into a microwave-safe measuring cup, combine the cocoa butter, oil, and beeswax. Stir.

3. In a microwave oven, heat the cup for 30 seconds on high. The mixture will be hot! Stir.

4. If the cocoa butter and beeswax are melted, you're ready to pour. If not melted, heat the mixture in 10-second intervals, until fully melted.

5. Pour the mixture into the PVC mold until it completely fills the sphere with a little "dome" on top. (If you overfill, you can wipe off the excess after it cools.)

6. Wait 30 seconds, then place the insert and bottom onto the top of the melted ingredients. Let the wax harden for 25 minutes. (If you want to speed up the process, place the mold in the freezer.)

7. Gently press on the dimple in the mold to set the balm firmly into the insert. (If balm spilled over the edge when you were filling the mold, now is the time to wipe it off with a tissue.)

8. Rub your lip balm creation onto your lips! Remember to discard any unused balm after two months.

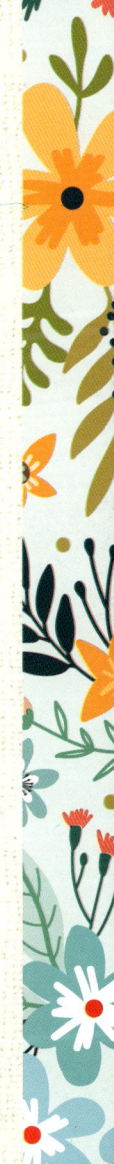

Cocoa Butter Kisses Lip Balm

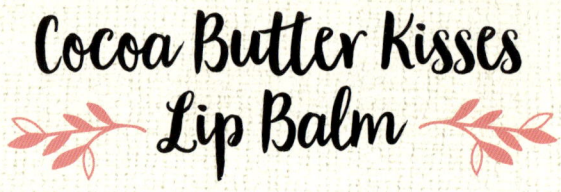

Made from the cocoa bean, cocoa butter is one of the key ingredients in chocolate. It blends easily when warm and solidifies at room temperature, making it ideal to use in chocolate manufacturing. The cocoa butter in this lip balm comes from actual chocolate candy, doing double time as an emollient and as a delicious flavoring.

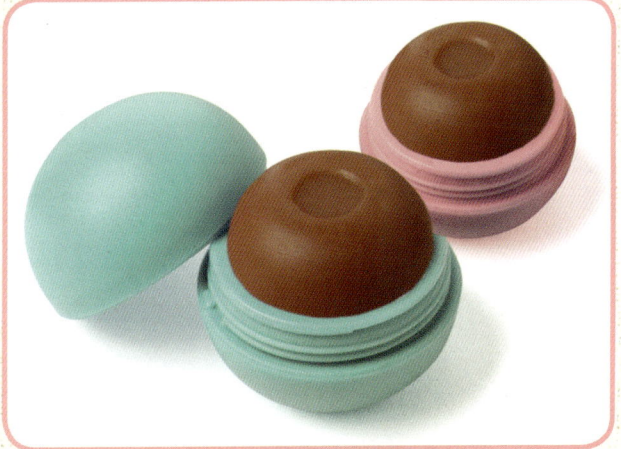

INGREDIENTS

1 teaspoon (5 mL) oil

1/2 teaspoon (2.5 mL) beeswax pastilles

2 chocolate chips

TOOLS

Microwave-safe measuring cup

Measuring spoons

Stir stick

PVC mold (from this kit)

Pod with insert (from this kit)

MAKES ONE LIP BALM

INSTRUCTIONS

1. Into a microwave-safe measuring cup, combine the oil and beeswax. Stir.

2. In a microwave oven, heat the cup for 30 seconds on high. The mixture will be hot! Stir. If the beeswax is not melted, heat the mixture in 10-second intervals, until fully melted.

3. Add the chocolate, and stir until incorporated.

4. Pour the mixture into the PVC mold until it completely fills the sphere with a little "dome" on top. (If you overfill, you can wipe off the excess after it cools.)

5. Wait 30 seconds, then place the insert and bottom onto the top of the melted ingredients. Let the wax harden for 25 minutes. (If you want to speed up the process, place the mold in the freezer.)

6. Gently press on the dimple in the mold to set the balm firmly into the insert. (If balm spilled over the edge when you were filling the mold, now is the time to wipe it off with a tissue.)

7. Rub your lip balm creation onto your lips! And remember to discard any unused balm after two months.

> You can replace the chocolate chips with 1/3 of a chocolate kiss or dark chocolate. The richer the taste, the less you'll need to create the perfect lip balm!

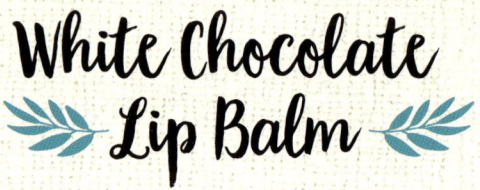

White Chocolate Lip Balm

Debates abound over whether or not white chocolate is indeed chocolate. It is missing a key ingredient: cocoa. However, it still includes the emollient properties of all chocolate due to one of its main ingredients: cocoa butter. So if you're a fan of this sweet treat, never mind its dubious status, and try this simple recipe.

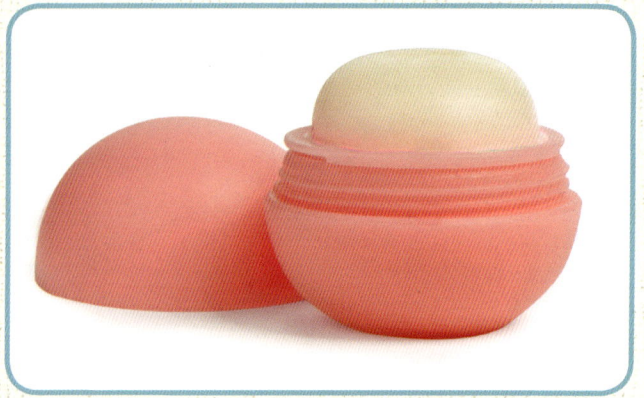

INGREDIENTS

1 teaspoon (5 mL) oil
1/2 teaspoon (2.5 mL) beeswax
  pastilles
2 white chocolate chips

TOOLS

Microwave-safe measuring cup
Measuring spoons
Stir stick
PVC mold (from this kit)
Pod with insert (from this kit)

MAKES ONE LIP BALM

INSTRUCTIONS

1. Into a microwave-safe measuring cup, combine the oil and beeswax. Stir.

2. In a microwave oven, heat the cup for 30 seconds on high. The mixture will be hot! If the beeswax is not melted, heat the mixture in 10-second intervals, until fully melted.

3. Add the white chocolate, and stir until incorporated.

4. Pour the mixture into the PVC mold until it completely fills the sphere with a little "dome" on top. (If you overfill, you can wipe off the excess after it cools.)

5. Wait 30 seconds, then place the insert and bottom onto the top of the melted ingredients. Let the wax harden for 25 minutes. (If you want to speed up the process, place the mold in the freezer.)

6. Gently press on the dimple in the mold to set the balm firmly into the insert. (If balm spilled over the edge when you were filling the mold, now is the time to wipe it off with a tissue.)

7. Rub your lip balm creation onto your lips! Remember to discard any unused balm after two months.

> To experience the full chocolate spectrum, experiment with milk chocolate and semi-sweet chocolate chips. Or for a whole new flavor, try butterscotch chips.

Chocolate Deluxe Lip Balm

The splurge-worthy ingredients in this rich lip balm are coconut oil and cocoa butter but chocolate's no slacker. Common knowledge tells us that chocolate can improve our mood by stimulating the production of our pleasure-stimulating endorphins. And dark chocolate even includes a compound that, among a laundry list of other benefits, can improve skin's hydration. Chocolate's only con might be its calorie count—not an issue with this recipe!

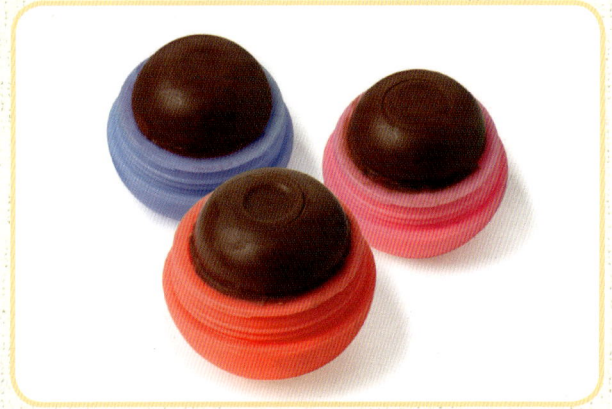

INGREDIENTS

1/2 teaspoon (2.5 mL) cocoa butter
1/2 teaspoon (2.5 mL) virgin coconut oil
1/2 teaspoon (2.5 mL) beeswax pastilles
Vitamin E (one or two capsules)
4 chocolate chips

TOOLS

Grater or chef's knife
Microwave-safe measuring cup
Measuring spoons
Stir stick
PVC mold (from this kit)
Pod with insert (from this kit)

MAKES ONE LIP BALM

INSTRUCTIONS

1. Grate or chop the cocoa butter into small pieces.

2. Into a microwave-safe measuring cup, combine the cocoa butter, coconut oil, and beeswax. Stir.

3. In a microwave oven, heat the cup for 30 seconds on high. The mixture will be hot! Stir. If the beeswax is not melted, heat the mixture in 10-second intervals, until fully melted.

4. Add the chocolate, and stir until incorporated.

5. Pour the mixture into the PVC mold until it completely fills the sphere with a little "dome" on top. (If you overfill, you can wipe off the excess after it cools.)

6. Wait 30 seconds, then place the insert and bottom onto the top of the melted ingredients. Let the wax harden for 25 minutes. (If you want to speed up the process, place the mold in the freezer.)

7. Gently press on the dimple in the mold to set the balm firmly into the insert. (If balm spilled over the edge when you were filling the mold, now is the time to wipe it off with a tissue.)

8. Rub your lip balm creation onto your lips! Remember to discard any unused balm after two months.

Honey Vanilla Lip Balm

Mixed with vanilla, this sweet-smelling lip balm packs the healing power of honey. A natural humectant, honey moisturizes and heals dry, chapped lips. And, because honey also has antibacterial qualities, it helps prevent infection from developing in those sore lips.

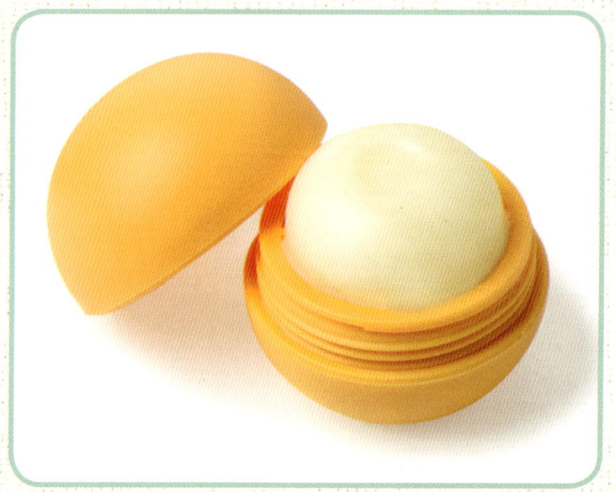

INGREDIENTS

1 teaspoon (5 mL) oil

1/2 teaspoon (2.5 mL) beeswax pastilles

1 drop honey

1 drop vanilla extract

TOOLS

Microwave-safe measuring cup

Measuring spoons

Stir stick

PVC mold (from this kit)

Pod with insert (from this kit)

MAKES ONE LIP BALM

INSTRUCTIONS

1. Into a microwave-safe measuring cup, combine the oil and beeswax. Stir.

2. In a microwave oven, heat the cup for 30 seconds on high. The mixture will be hot! Stir. If the beeswax is not melted, heat the mixture in 10-second intervals, until fully melted.

3. Let the mixture cool a bit. Then add the honey and vanilla, and stir briskly. It will take a lot of mixing to get the add-ins to blend with the oil.

4. Pour the mixture into the PVC mold, and keep stirring until the ingredients start to harden. Be sure to it completely fill the sphere with a little "dome" on top. (If you overfill, you can wipe off the excess after it cools.)

5. Wait 30 seconds, then place the insert and bottom onto the top of the melted ingredients. Let the wax harden for 25 minutes. (If you want to speed up the process, place the mold in the freezer.)

6. Gently press on the dimple in the mold to set the balm firmly into the insert. (If balm spilled over the edge when you were filling the mold, now is the time to wipe it off with a tissue.)

7. Rub your lip balm creation onto your lips! Remember to discard any unused balm after two months.

> Use sweet almond oil for the oil in this recipe and skip the vanilla.

Orange Cream Layered Lip Balm

Layer things up with a summertime-themed lip balm. Start with this simple vanilla and orange cream recipe to get the hang of it. Then switch up your stripes—any variation of color or flavoring can be achieved with these directions. Once you've perfected the technique, try making multiple layers of two different colors. Or three!

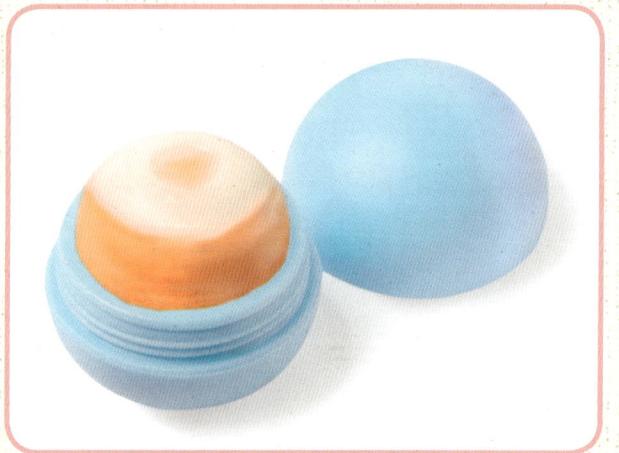

INGREDIENTS

1 teaspoon (5 mL) oil
1/2 teaspoon (2.5 mL) beeswax pastilles
1/2 orange candy melt
1 to 2 drops orange flavoring oil

TOOLS

Microwave-safe measuring cup
Measuring spoons
Stir stick
PVC mold (from this kit)
Pod with insert (from this kit)

MAKES ONE LIP BALM

INSTRUCTIONS

1. Into a microwave-safe measuring cup, combine the oil and beeswax. Stir.

2. In a microwave oven, heat the cup for 30 seconds on high. The mixture will be hot! Stir. If the beeswax is melted, you're ready to pour. If the beeswax is not melted, heat the mixture in 10-second intervals, until fully melted.

3. Pour a little less than half of the mixture into the PVC mold.

4. Into the remaining melted oil, add the orange candy melt. Stir well to mix in the color. You may need to reheat it for a few seconds. If so, heat at 5-second intervals until everything is melted. Add the orange flavoring oil, and stir until incorporated.

5. When a white skin has formed on top of the mixture in the mold (about 1 minute), carefully pour the colored mixture on top until it completely fills the sphere with a little "dome" on top. If you overfill, you can wipe off the excess after it cools.

6. Wait 30 seconds, then place the insert and bottom onto the top of the melted ingredients. Let the wax harden for 25 minutes. (If you want to speed up the process, place the mold in the freezer.)

7. Gently press on the dimple in the mold to set the balm firmly into the insert. (If balm spilled over the edge when you were filling the mold, now is the time to wipe it off with a tissue.)

8. Rub your lip balm creation onto your lips! Remember to discard any unused balm after two months.

Try your hand at three layers inspired by another cool treat: Neapolitan ice cream!

Cherry Bomb
Lip Balm

Cherries are full of powerful antioxidants. Some varieties are purported to be superior even to vitamin E, which is known to calm your skin and help protect it from sun damage. This cherry lip balm is colored and flavored to appear cherry-like so follow nature's cue and add in vitamin E to elevate your benefits! Just use a toothpick to poke a hole in a vitamin E capsule, and then squeeze out the oil!

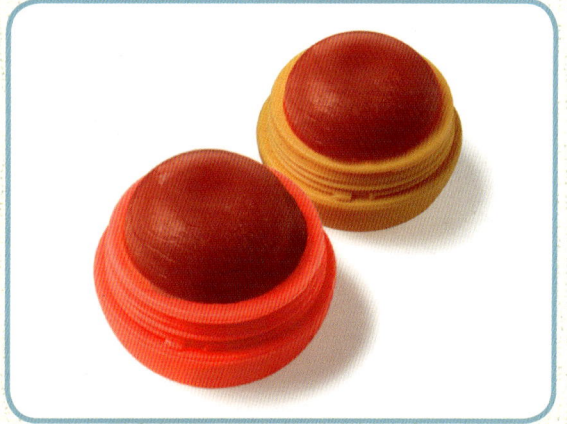

INGREDIENTS

1/2 teaspoon (2.5 mL) oil

1/2 teaspoon (2.5 mL) beeswax
   pastilles

1 red candy melt

Vitamin E (oil from 1 to 2
   capsules)

1 to 2 drops cherry flavoring oil

TOOLS

Microwave-safe measuring cup

Measuring spoons

Stir stick

PVC mold (from this kit)

Pod with insert (from this kit)

MAKES ONE LIP BALM

INSTRUCTIONS

1. Into a microwave-safe measuring cup, combine the oil and beeswax. Stir.

2. In a microwave oven, heat the cup for 30 seconds on high. The mixture will be hot! Stir. If the beeswax is not melted, heat the mixture in 10-second intervals, until fully melted.

3. Add the candy melt, vitamin E, and flavoring oil. Stir until incorporated.

4. Pour the mixture into the PVC mold until it completely fills the sphere with a little "dome" on top. (If you overfill, you can wipe off the excess after it cools.)

5. Wait 30 seconds, then place the insert and bottom onto the top of the melted ingredients. Let the wax harden for 25 minutes. (If you want to speed up the process, place the mold in the freezer.)

6. Gently press on the dimple in the mold to set the balm firmly into the insert. (If balm spilled over the edge when you were filling the mold, now is the time to wipe it off with a tissue.)

7. Rub your lip balm creation onto your lips! Remember to discard any unused balm after two months.

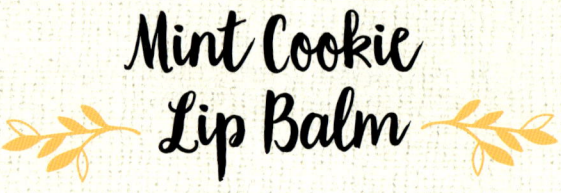

Mint Cookie Lip Balm

Maybe it's not Girl Scout cookie season and your freezer is empty of your stockpile of favorite snacks. This recipe can help tide you over. True peppermint oil is a medicinal treatment that's been around since Cleopatra's day. Breathe deep and receive the benefits that mint's scent has to offer, not the least of which is to ease stress.

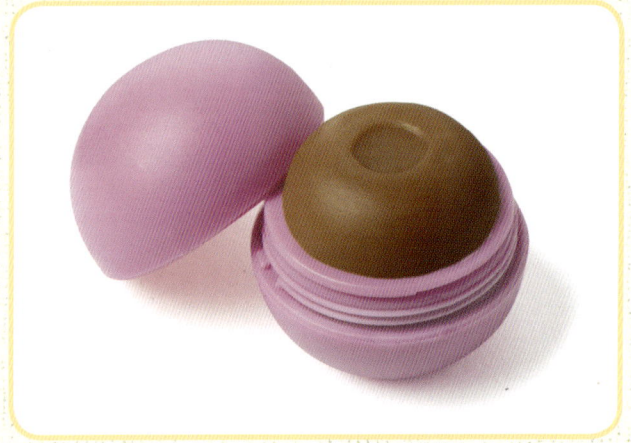

INGREDIENTS

1 teaspoon (5 mL) oil

1/2 teaspoon (2.5 mL) beeswax pastilles

2 chocolate chips

1 to 2 drops peppermint flavoring oil

TOOLS

Microwave-safe measuring cup

Measuring spoons

Stir stick

PVC mold (from this kit)

Pod with insert (from this kit)

MAKES ONE LIP BALM

INSTRUCTIONS

1. Into a microwave-safe measuring cup, combine the oil and beeswax. Stir.

2. In a microwave oven, heat the cup for 30 seconds on high. The mixture will be hot! Stir. If the beeswax is not melted, heat the mixture in 10-second intervals, until fully melted.

3. Add the chocolate chips and flavoring oil. Stir until incorporated.

4. Pour the mixture into the PVC mold until it completely fills the sphere with a little "dome" on top. (If you overfill, you can wipe off the excess after it cools.)

5. Wait 30 seconds, then place the insert and bottom onto the top of the melted ingredients. Let the wax harden for 25 minutes. (If you want to speed up the process, place the mold in the freezer.)

6. Gently press on the dimple in the mold to set the balm firmly into the insert. (If balm spilled over the edge when you were filling the mold, now is the time to wipe it off with a tissue.)

7. Rub your lip balm creation onto your lips! Remember to discard any unused balm after two months.

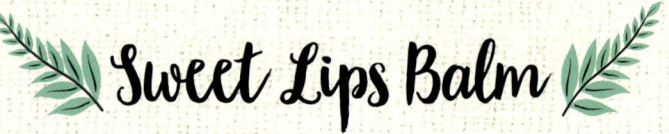

Sweet Lips Balm

Candy melts give your balms a hint of flavor (typically vanilla) and come in myriad colors. For this lip balm, choose your favorite. Sugar doesn't get much love in the "good for you" category but in this small dose, it doesn't have to be a big deal.

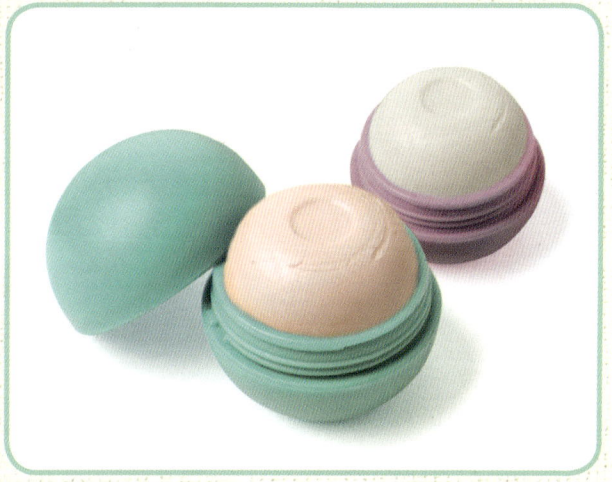

INGREDIENTS

1 teaspoon (5 mL) oil

1/2 teaspoon (2.5 mL) beeswax pastilles

1 candy melt (color of your choice)

TOOLS

Microwave-safe measuring cup

Measuring spoons

Stir stick

PVC mold (from this kit)

Pod with insert (from this kit)

MAKES ONE LIP BALM

INSTRUCTIONS

1. Into a microwave-safe measuring cup, combine the oil and beeswax. Stir.

2. In a microwave oven, heat the cup for 30 seconds on high. Mixture will be hot! Stir. If the beeswax is not melted, heat the mixture in 10-second intervals, until fully melted.

3. Add the candy melt, and stir until incorporated.

4. Pour the mixture into the PVC mold until it completely fills the sphere with a little "dome" on top. (If you overfill, you can wipe off the excess after it cools.)

5. Wait 30 seconds, then place the insert and bottom onto the top of the melted ingredients. Let the wax harden for 25 minutes. (If you want to speed up the process, place the mold in the freezer.)

6. Gently press on the dimple in the mold to set the balm firmly into the insert. (If balm spilled over the edge when you were filling the mold, now is the time to wipe it off with a tissue.)

7. Rub your lip balm creation onto your lips! Remember to discard any unused balm after two months.

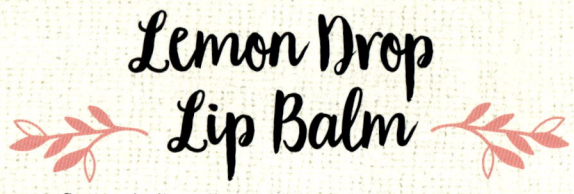

Lemon Drop Lip Balm

Use lemon-flavored olive oil to add the light scent of fresh lemons to this lip balm. Simply replace the oil you've been using in your standard recipe to this specialty oil. Even without the citrus addition, olive oil often possesses a deeper color and a fruitier flavor than other oils. Better yet, it's packed with antioxidants so it protects your skin, keeping it healthy.

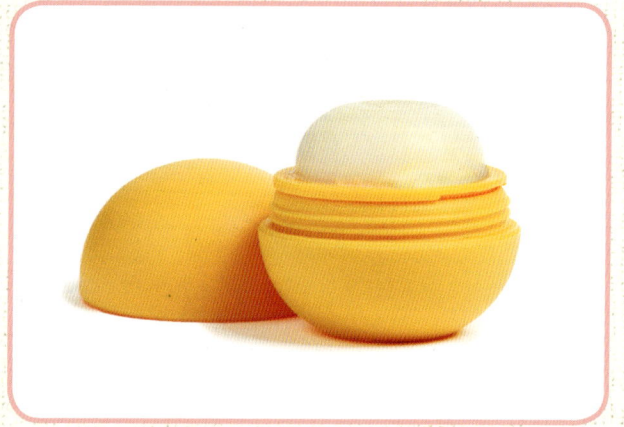

INGREDIENTS

1 teaspoon (5 mL) lemon-flavored olive oil

1/2 teaspoon (2.5 mL) beeswax pastilles

TOOLS

Microwave-safe measuring cup

Measuring spoons

Stir stick

PVC mold (from this kit)

Pod with insert (from this kit)

MAKES ONE LIP BALM

INSTRUCTIONS

1. Into a microwave-safe measuring cup, combine the oil and beeswax. Stir.

2. In a microwave oven, heat the cup for 30 seconds on high. Mixture will be hot! Stir. If the beeswax is melted, you're ready to pour. If the beeswax is not melted, heat the mixture in 10-second intervals, until fully melted.

3. Pour the mixture into the PVC mold until it completely fills the sphere with a little "dome" on top. (If you overfill, you can wipe off the excess after it cools.)

4. Wait 30 seconds, then place the insert and bottom onto the top of the melted ingredients. Let the wax harden for 25 minutes. (If you want to speed up the process, place the mold in the freezer.)

5. Gently press on the dimple in the mold to set the balm firmly into the insert. (If balm spilled over the edge when you were filling the mold, now is the time to wipe it off with a tissue.)

6. Rub your lip balm creation onto your lips! Remember to discard any unused balm after two months.

Chocolate Hazelnut Lip Balm

In an effort to extend his chocolate, and likely his livelihood, an Italian chocolatier mixed hazelnuts into his confections as a reaction to the scarcity—and expense—of chocolate during the Napoleonic era. Stretching his supply spawned what's become an incredibly popular and beloved chocolate-hazelnut spread. Boost your lip balm's effectiveness with the special add-in of glycerin. A by-product of soapmaking, it is a humectant so it attracts water, which helps keep your lips from drying out.

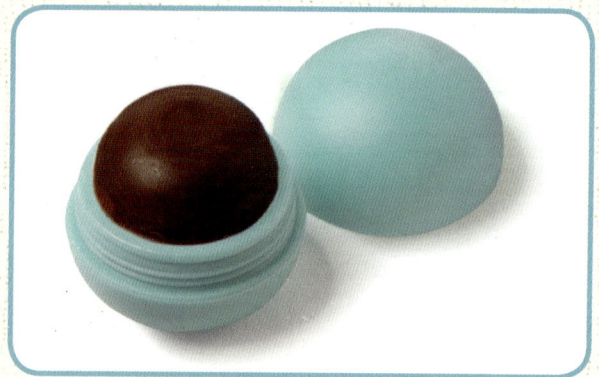

INGREDIENTS

1 teaspoon (5 mL) oil

1/2 teaspoon (2.5 mL) beeswax pastilles

1 teaspoon (5mL) of chocolate hazelnut spread

2 drops liquid glycerin (optional)

TOOLS

Microwave-safe measuring cup

Measuring spoons

Stir stick

PVC mold (from this kit)

Pod with insert (from this kit)

MAKES ONE LIP BALM

INSTRUCTIONS

1. Into a microwave-safe measuring cup, combine the oil and beeswax. Stir.

2. In a microwave oven, heat the cup for 30 seconds on high. Mixture will be hot! Stir. If the beeswax is not melted, heat the mixture in 10-second intervals, until fully melted.

3. Add the chocolate-hazelnut spread and glycerin. Stir until incorporated.

4. Pour the mixture into the PVC mold until it completely fills the sphere with a little "dome" on top. (If you overfill, you can wipe off the excess after it cools.)

5. Wait 30 seconds, then place the insert and bottom onto the top of the melted ingredients. Let the wax harden for 25 minutes. (If you want to speed up the process, place the mold in the freezer.)

6. Gently press on the dimple in the mold to set the balm firmly into the insert. (If balm spilled over the edge when you were filling the mold, now is the time to wipe it off with a tissue.)

7. Rub your lip balm creation onto your lips! Remember to discard any unused balm after two months.

Pretty and Pink

For a whisper of color, mix some shavings of your favorite—or forgotten—lipstick into the base ingredients of this lip balm recipe. Pale, unscented castor oil conditions lips and, due to its thick consistency, increases the gloss factor in this tinted lip balm. It'll stay on your lips longer too. Bonus: Castor oil inhibits the growth of bacteria. (It's still a good idea to dispose of any lip balm that's more than two months old.)

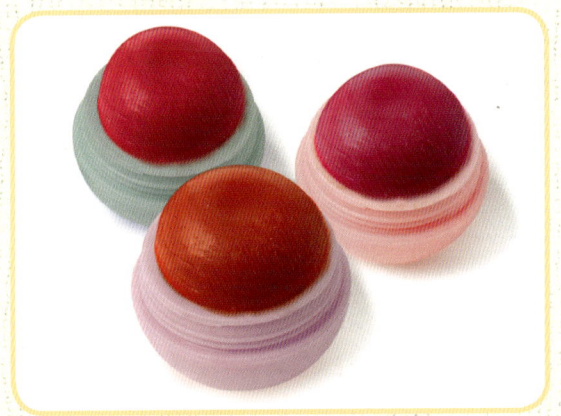

INGREDIENTS

1/2 teaspoon (2.5 mL) oil

1/2 teaspoon (2.5 mL) beeswax pastilles

Lipstick shavings

2 to 3 drops castor oil

TOOLS

Microwave-safe measuring cup

Measuring spoons

Stir stick

PVC mold (from this kit)

Pod with insert (from this kit)

MAKES ONE LIP BALM

INSTRUCTIONS

1. Into a microwave-safe measuring cup, combine the beeswax and oil. Stir.

2. In a microwave oven, heat the cup for 30 seconds on high. The mixture will be hot! Stir. If the beeswax is not melted, heat the mixture in 10-second intervals, until fully melted.

3. Add the lipstick shavings and castor oil. Stir until incorporated.

4. Pour the mixture into the PVC mold until it completely fills the sphere with a little "dome" on top. If you overfill, you can wipe off the excess after it cools.

5. Wait 30 seconds, then place the insert and bottom onto the top of the melted ingredients. Let the wax harden for 25 minutes. (If you want to speed up the process, place the mold in the freezer.)

6. Gently press on the dimple in the mold to set the balm firmly into the insert. (If balm spilled over the edge when you were filling the mold, now is the time to wipe it off with a tissue.)

7. Rub your lip balm creation onto your lips! Remember to discard any unused balm after two months.

Shimmering Frost Lip Balm

Once upon a time, you entered the kitchen determined to elevate your beauty products to a homemade, handcrafted level. You scoured your pantry, organized your ingredients, and pushed the limits of natural beauty, inspired to intentionally make blue lip balm with the shimmery addition of cosmetic-grade glitter you found online.

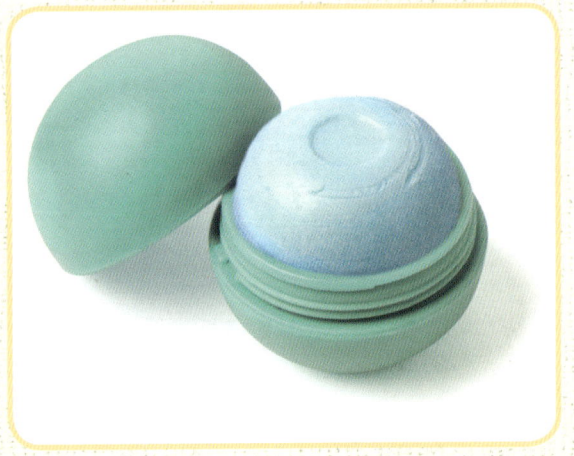

INGREDIENTS

1 teaspoon (5 mL) oil

1/2 teaspoon (2.5 mL) beeswax pastilles

1 bright white candy melt

1/2 blue candy melt

2 drops peppermint oil (optional)

Cosmetic-grade glitter (optional)

TOOLS

Microwave-safe measuring cup

Measuring spoons

Stir stick

PVC mold (from this kit)

Pod with insert (from this kit)

MAKES ONE LIP BALM

INSTRUCTIONS

1. Into a microwave-safe measuring cup, combine the beeswax and oil. Stir.

2. In a microwave oven, heat the cup for 30 seconds on high. The mixture will be hot! Stir. If the beeswax is melted, you're ready to pour. If the beeswax is not melted, heat the mixture in 10-second intervals, until fully melted.

3. Add both candy melts, and stir until incorporated. Blend in the peppermint oil and glitter.

4. Pour the mixture into the PVC mold until it completely fills the sphere with a little "dome" on top. If you overfill, you can wipe off the excess after it cools.

5. Wait 30 seconds, then place the insert and bottom onto the top of the melted ingredients. Let the wax harden for 25 minutes. (If you want to speed up the process, place the mold in the freezer.)

6. Gently press on the dimple in the mold to set the balm firmly into the insert. (If balm spilled over the edge when you were filling the mold, now is the time to wipe it off with a tissue.)

7. Rub your lip balm creation onto your lips! Remember to discard any unused balm after two months.

Beyond Lip Balm:

Because the skin on your lips is very thin compared to the rest of the skin on your face, your lips need extra protection. Keep them in top shape by exfoliating with one of these sugary scrubs to reveal fresh skin.

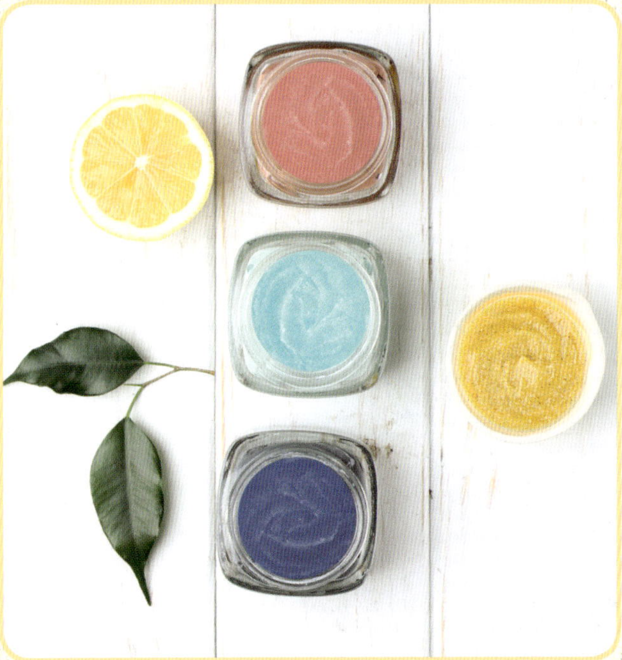

Simple Sugar Scrubs

Sugar's natural humectant properties make the sugar scrubs a more hydrating proposition than its better-known cousin, the salt scrub. Its smaller granule makes it gentler to the skin too. And in this case—applying it to the lips—it's going to taste better!

INGREDIENTS

1/2 tsp (2.5 mL) sugar
1/2 tsp (2.5 mL) honey
2 to 3 drops olive oil

TOOLS

Small bowl
Stir stick

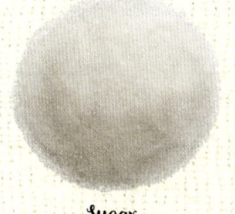

Sugar

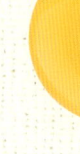

Honey

Olive oil

MAKES ENOUGH FOR ONE APPLICATION

INSTRUCTIONS

1. Into a small bowl, measure out the sugar, honey, and olive oil. Stir to make a paste.

2. Apply the mixture to your lips and gently buff with your fingers for about 1 minute.

3. Rinse off with a scrub of a toothbrush or washcloth for extra exfoliating power!

Brown Sugar Scrub

Brown sugar particles are even smaller than granulated sugar making this scrub the go-to for those with sensitive skin. It dissolves easily in water so rinses off quickly. And along with its companions, olive oil, honey, and vanilla, this all-natural brown sugar scrub smells amazing!

INGREDIENTS

1 teaspoon (5 mL) brown sugar
1/2 teaspoon (2.5 mL) olive oil
1/4 teaspoon (1 mL) honey
2 drops vanilla extract

TOOLS

Small bowl
Stir stick

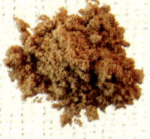   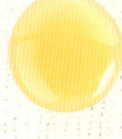 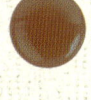

Brown sugar   Honey   Olive oil   Vanilla extract

MAKES ENOUGH FOR ONE APPLICATION

INSTRUCTIONS

1. Into a small bowl, measure out the brown sugar, olive oil, and honey. Stir to make a paste.

2. Apply the mixture to your lips and gently buff with your fingers for about 1 minute.

3. Rinse off with a scrub of a toothbrush or washcloth for extra exfoliating power!